Personal Healthcare Record

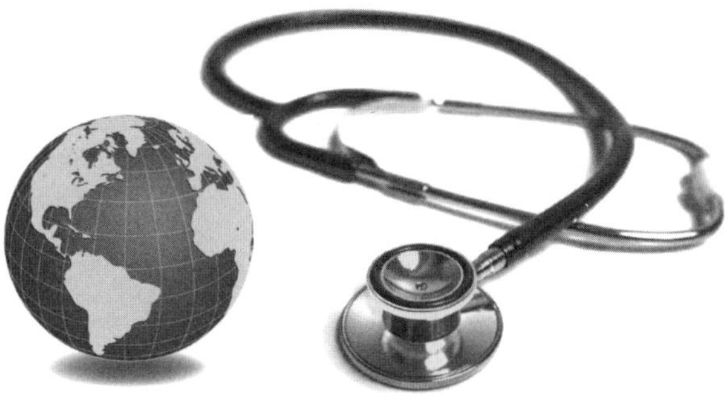

Adult

For ______________________________
Name

From ____________ *to* ____________
Date *Date*

CONFIDENTIAL

Don't Forget

Tortuga Publishing, 2011

A Division of Tortuga Enterprises LLC

A request from the author: *I have developed this journal at the lowest possible cost for the user. While it may be tempting to photocopy this entire record to share with others, I am appealing to your basic sense of honesty and compliance with copyright law to refrain from reproducing or otherwise providing copies of the contents to others. You may reproduce, for your personal use, the template pages (additional journal pages, spine and cover for additional notebooks for your own records).*
Thank you for your purchase,
Charla Hornung Spence

To buy additional copies or send comments, visit our website:

Website: www.PersonalHealthcareRecord.com

First Printing, 2011

Library of Congrees Control Number: 2009942076

ISBN: 978-0-9744643-4-3

Tortuga Publishing
A Division of Tortuga Enterprises LLC
1142 S. Diamond Bar #261
CA 91765
United States of America

What they're saying....

"This is a vital gift for every new baby from every grandparent!" And adult children can do the same for their older adults whose healthcare gets more complicated every year. I especially appreciated the history charts—I am always filling them out, but forgetting the years and other details."
Kathleen L., Grandmother, Bellingham, WA

"...this would be a great tool for a parent to start for a child...As I fill out medical forms, I realize I can't recall exact dates and details of previous health conditions or treatments. Having everything in one location...trying to remember everything...this could have made everything so much easier. "
Shelley F., Baby Boomer, Phoenix, AZ

"The PHR finally motivated me to get my medical life in order. The thought of organizing my health records was daunting until I saw how the PHR did most of the work for me—add a few notes, staple some doctor's info. together and I was done! And it has been fun to track, which is easy now that all the info. is in one place."
Bill H., Carlsbad, CA

"We've all heard encouraging messages like 'take charge of your own healthcare or be a part of your healthcare team,' sending the message loud and clear that the most important person on your healthcare team is YOU! This PHR is the right tool for doing that! It's a means for organizing your healthcare information to keep you in charge—helping you connect the dots. There was a time when we could rely on doctors to do that; those days are gone."
Joseph S., Healthcare Consultant, South Jordan, UT

"The PHR is a valuable tool for everyone, ESPECIALLY in an emergency. Under extreme circumstances, time and proper diagnosis can make the difference between life and death. The ability to quickly access vital information from the patient, family member or caretaker can expedite the diagnosis process, saving valuable time. In a non-emergency situation, information is often lost in translation. A doctor's ability to treat is dependent on the history of the patient. Having the ability to view previous tests often eliminates the need to duplicate some tests. It also gives the physician a baseline for referencing changes in the patient's condition. I love my PHR and my family endorses it as well. Thanks!"
Susan C., CRT, Alta Loma, CA

"Most people struggle to remember symptoms and how they evolved over the course of treatment. Providing a tool that helps people be more disciplined about this process is a valuable service. Thank you!"
Susan H., Consultant, Oakland, CA

The Author's Story

The genesis for this journal came from a personal need. Over the past several years, I have faced a number of medical issues personally and within my family. To mention just a few, my mother was diagnosed with cancer and eventually passed away from Alzheimer's disease; my father had heart value replacement and a gangrenous gall bladder removed; my daughter incurred a serious neck injury, my sister was diagnosed and succumbed to cancer. My husband passed away unexpectedly from complications of a common surgery. His PHR was valuable in analyzing medical issues related to his death. I've had several medical situations that have led to surgeries and other treatments. It soon became very evident that a user-friendly system for organizing all these converging events was greatly needed. So, I began organizing all of our medical information to make it easier to keep everything and everyone's situations straight.

Along the way, I came to the conclusion that it made sense to begin this record at birth rather than in later life. While it's never too late to begin gathering and maintaining healthcare information, doing so earlier makes the information easier to collect and keep complete.

My initial efforts eventually inspired me to develop the this tool. I know that if you use this journal as intended, you will find it valuable too.

Take charge of your healthcare and best wishes for a long and healthy life!

Charla Hornung Spence

Dedication

To my husband, my mother and sister, Sally, now living with the angels.

Acknowledgements

Just as it takes a village to raise a child, it takes a team to publish a book. The PHR was truly a team effort and I must thank many for helping me develop this tool into something that will help people begin taking charge of their healthcare. I thank the healthcare professionals who evaluated and provided valuable input, particularly: Holly Ferguson, Physician Assistant; Susan Cuzynski, CRT. End-user consultants: Susan Harris, Bill Hornung, Joseph Stith, Shelley and John Fletcher, Kathleen Whiteside Langdon. I also thank Michael Adams who provided developmental critiques and editing services.; Antoinette and Jared Kurtiz, Strategies Literary Public Relations for their guidance and support in the publishing and marketing process; Lloyd Jassin for legal counsel; Gwyn Kennedy Snider for graphics; Meredith Gould for copy editing; and Brian Jud, Greg Snider and Amy Collins MacGregor for supporting distribution.

I wish to thank the Southern California Writers Association for their great industry speakers and much more. In my role as Secretary and Vice President of Membership, I have forged many friendships for which I am grateful.

I thank my family for their inspiration and support—my parents Charlotte and Bill, brother Bill, sister Lanna, husband Michael, daughter Jessica, and other family members and friends.

Contents

The contents of your Personal Healthcare Record are not designed to replace your doctors' healthcare advice or records. The PHR is intended to serve as an organizational aide only.

Foreword

Given the realities of today's healthcare and health insurance world, your will likely have several different doctors, each of whom specialize in the treatment of any condition you might develop. A Personal Healthcare Record (PHR) will help you navigate the healthcare terrain by providing important background and baseline information for the healthcare professionals you will visit. Maintained carefully and well, a PHR will help you prevent taking a lot of unnecessary or redundant steps that may cost money or, at the very least, time.

Charla Spence is the perfect person to develop the PHR because she is not a healthcare professional. She's a patient just like you who recognized the need for this valuable tool. She developed the PHR from the patient's point-of-view, using common terms to provide a practicable, portable organizational system for your healthcare history. Because this is not a medical reference book, only very basic medical information is included.

Introduction

Everyone should have a Personal Healthcare Record (PHR). Ideally, such an organizational system should begin at birth and be updated throughout your entire life. Many healthcare professionals and agencies encourage individuals to take charge of their health by following standard guidelines for diet, exercise, disease prevention and health maintenance. Now you have a handy, easy-to-use tool for tracking all this vital information!

Icons used in this book:

Hints: helps you get the most value out of your PHR

Caution: "must dos" to keep your PHR information up to date

Note: important information that will be helpful to others

Benefits of keeping a PHR...

- READY-TO- GO The PHR reduces the thinking and time required for organizing this important information. Fill in the blanks, punch a few holes, and you're ready to go!
- PORTABLE This portable journal is easy to keep and transport. No need to access a computer or find the right software. No extra steps for entering constantly changing healthcare information. Add reports and comments on the spot! Sometimes the best technology is low technology!
- PERSONAL & FAMILY HISTORY When it's time for them to take responsibility for their own healthcare and records, hand your children their PHR and they'll have all of their healthcare history to date.
- CAREGIVER REFERENCE Relying on others to help care for your loved one? Trusted caregivers and family members can have healthcare records, along with the Advance Directive, in case the need arises.
- IN CASE OF EMERGENCY In an emergency, any trusted person can grab your PHR and use it to answer all the inevitable questions. In the case of a natural disaster, computers may not work. Grab your PHR & have everything you will need!

Note: *Make sure several trusted friends or family members know where you keep your PHR.*

How to Use This Journal

The PHR can be used in the bound book form; however, the PHR was developed for use in a 3-ring notebook format so that you can easily include additional pages, copies of medical tests, reports, etc. It also makes it easy to rearrange or move older documents to additional notebooks over time. The Healthcare History section and recent Journal pages should remain in the primary binder for easy reference by your healthcare providers, but since this is your journal feel free to rearrange it in whatever order makes sense to you. The icons are intended to draw your attention to important hints, notes or cautions.

Setting Up Your PHR

- ✓ Remove the perforated pages, hole punch and place the contents in a 3-ring notebook. You may want to purchase a view type binder so you can put the covers and spine in the slip covers provided on the outside of the notebook.
- ✓ Insert tab dividers and pocket folders based on preference. These can be purchased at any office supply store.
- ✓ Carry a hole punch to make it easy to add, on the spot, any documents received from healthcare providers. Convenient notebook size three hole punches can be purchased from any office supply store.

Hint: *Remember to keep all information in chronological (by the date) order to make it easy to reference. After setting up, move the Table of Contents and Introduction to the reference section.*

5 Simple Steps

To get the most from your PHR, please read and follow these 5 Simple Steps to get started.

1. Complete Healthcare History

Use Section B to capture information from the various healthcare sources as it becomes relevant and available. Work with your healthcare professionals to consolidate all healthcare history and other important information in one convenient place.

Caution! *You must update the PHR with any new information when you get it.*

Note: *Put Healthcare History at a Glance page in a page protector and make it the first page so that emergency personnel may find it quickly. Remove the wallet card page, cut to size indicated, complete information and place in your wallet for quick reference. Keep the wallet card in the template section so you can make new copies for future use.*

2. Prepare Journal Pages

Note or staple any new information from office visits and other updates onto your personal journal pages. Better yet, take the journal pages with you to make notes during each visit or other activity.

Even if you do not have a healthcare appointment scheduled, you can begin to prepare for that event by collecting Concerns/Questions/Symptoms to discuss with your healthcare professional and then, note them on a journal page. Most healthcare professionals do appreciate serving patients who come prepared with a list of questions. Not only does this make the appointment time more efficient, but it will help you ensure that all your concerns and questions are addressed. There's also space on each Journal page to record vital signs. The following is a key for the vital signs on the Journal page:

Journal Key:	BP – Blood Pressure	Gl – Glucose
	Ch – Cholesterol	Rp – Respirations
	HR – Heart Rate/Pulse	Tp – Temperature
	Ht – Height	Wt – Weight

Here are a few suggestions for making your visits to your healthcare professional more effective:

✓ Complete your PHR Journal page in advance of your appointment and take your PHR notebook with you. (See sample Journal Page on page 102)

Hint: *If you're returning to one of your regular doctors, you may want to take only the current journal page, in a folder for privacy, rather than carry the entire PHR. This will also reduce the chances of losing your PHR or a stranger seeing confidential information.*

✓ When making your appointment, let the appointment desk receptionist know if you have several items to discuss with the doctor in addition to the primary reason for your appointment.

✓ Write down all information and actions from your visit on the Journal page.

Hint: *You may prefer recording some of the information (like dental, hearing, vision or hospitalizations) on the optional pages 89-92 for quick reference and so that you do not have to dig for the information in the regular Journal pages.*

✓ If you use your PHR in the notebook format, insert an extra page behind any forms where additional space is needed. Make extra copies of the general use page titled Symptom/Healthcare Event Journal located in the template section for this purpose.

Caution: *Replace the Journal page and any related documents in the binder after your appointment so that the information is not misplaced.*

Note: *A convenient way for caregivers to help those who may attend appointments, with those being assisted, is to provide a list of questions on the journal page or insert an extra page with questions. Ask the healthcare professional to respond to the questions by writing answers directly on the journal page for your later reference.*

Remember, the ability for healthcare professionals to care of you is only as good as your ability to provide accurate information!

3. Record Appointment Information

As soon as possible after your appointment, or preferably during the appointment, complete the Journal page with Diagnosis, Actions Needed and Outcome. This will enhance your ability to follow through on any actions you may need to take. If you need additional room to record the information from the visit, insert another page, or use another journal section to write your comments.

Hint: *Be sure to get a business card from healthcare professionals so you have all of their contact information. You may attach the business card or write the information on the Journal page in the box provided.*

4. Punch and Insert Materials

You will likely receive all types of reports and test results in different sizes. Rather than take the extra time to scan into an electronic system, simply punch holes in the document, place it behind the appropriate appointment in the Journal pages and you're done!

Hint: *For ease of use, move completed Journal pages to the back of the Journal Section so next appointment page is on top. This will keep the pages in date order without getting in your way.*

5. Schedule Future Healthcare

Based on your healthcare professionals recommendations, schedule the routine appointments like annual physicals, dental, hearing and vision check-ups.

Hint: *When needed, photocopy additional Journal pages and wallet cards from templates in Reference Section C. Do not write on the templates so that you can continue to make additional copies.*

SECTION A

Journal Pages

Don't Forget

Personal Healthcare Record

Healthcare Concern/Questions/Symptoms

Date ____________

Staple physician's or other healthcare provider's business card or write in contact information here.

Referred by:

____

Include relevant vital sign measurements as medical personnel complete your evaluation. (Reference key on page xi.)

BP ________ HR________ Tp________ Rp________

HT________ Wt________ GL ________ Ch ________

Other ______________________________

Diagnosis

Actions Needed *(follow-up, referral, prescriptions, tests, etc.)* Date Scheduled

Outcome

Healthcare Concern/Questions/Symptoms

Date ____________

Staple physician's or other healthcare provider's business card or write in contact information here.

Referred by:

____

Diagnosis

Include relevant vital sign measurements as medical personnel complete your evaluation. (Reference key on page xi.)

BP ______ HR______ Tp______ Rp______

HT______ Wt______ GL______ Ch______

Other ______________________

Actions Needed *(follow-up, referral, prescriptions, tests, etc.)*

Date Scheduled

Outcome

Healthcare Concern/Questions/Symptoms

Date ____________

Staple physician's or other healthcare provider's business card or write in contact information here.

Referred by:

____

Include relevant vital sign measurements as medical personnel complete your evaluation. (Reference key on page xi.)

BP________ HR________ Tp________ Rp________

HT________ Wt________ GL________ Ch________

Other ______________________________

Diagnosis

Actions Needed *(follow-up, referral, prescriptions, tests, etc.)*

Date Scheduled

Outcome

Personal Healthcare Record for: ______________________ *Page* ________

Healthcare Concern/Questions/Symptoms

Date ____________

Staple physician's or other healthcare provider's business card or write in contact information here.

Referred by:

____

Include relevant vital sign measurements as medical personnel complete your evaluation. (Reference key on page xi.)

BP________ HR________ Tp________ Rp________

HT________ Wt________ GL________ Ch________

Other ____________________

Diagnosis

Actions Needed *(follow-up, referral, prescriptions, tests, etc.)*

Date Scheduled

Outcome

Personal Healthcare Record for: ______________________________ *Page* ________

Healthcare Concern/Questions/Symptoms

Date ____________

Staple physician's or other healthcare provider's business card or write in contact information here.

Referred by:

____

Include relevant vital sign measurements as medical personnel complete your evaluation. (Reference key on page xi.)

BP ________ HR________ Tp________ Rp________

HT________ Wt________ GL ________ Ch_______

Other ______________________________

Diagnosis

Actions Needed *(follow-up, referral, prescriptions, tests, etc.)*

Date Scheduled

Outcome

Healthcare Concern/Questions/Symptoms

Date ____________

Staple physician's or other healthcare provider's business card or write in contact information here.

Referred by:

____

Include relevant vital sign measurements as medical personnel complete your evaluation. (Reference key on page xi.)

BP ______ HR______ Tp______ Rp______

HT______ Wt______ GL______ Ch______

Other ____________________

Diagnosis

Actions Needed *(follow-up, referral, prescriptions, tests, etc.)*

Date Scheduled

Outcome

Healthcare Concern/Questions/Symptoms

Date ________

Staple physician's or other healthcare provider's business card or write in contact information here.

Referred by:

____

Diagnosis

Include relevant vital sign measurements as medical personnel complete your evaluation. (Reference key on page xi.)

BP ________ HR________ Tp________ Rp________

HT________ Wt________ GL ________ Ch ________

Other ____________________

Actions Needed *(follow-up, referral, prescriptions, tests, etc.)*

Date Scheduled

Outcome

Healthcare Concern/Questions/Symptoms

Date ____________

Staple physician's or other healthcare provider's business card or write in contact information here.

Referred by:

____

Include relevant vital sign measurements as medical personnel complete your evaluation. (Reference key on page xi.)

BP ________ HR________ Tp________ Rp________

HT ________ Wt________ GL ________ Ch ________

Other ______________________

Diagnosis

Actions Needed *(follow-up, referral, prescriptions, tests, etc.)* Date Scheduled

Outcome

Personal Healthcare Record for: ______________________________ *Page* ________

Healthcare Concern/Questions/Symptoms

Date ____________

Staple physician's or other healthcare provider's business card or write in contact information here.

Referred by:

____

Include relevant vital sign measurements as medical personnel complete your evaluation. (Reference key on page xi.)

BP ________ HR________ Tp________ Rp________

HT________ Wt________ GL ________ Ch________

Other ______________________________

Diagnosis

Actions Needed *(follow-up, referral, prescriptions, tests, etc.)*

Date Scheduled

Outcome

Healthcare Concern/Questions/Symptoms

Date ____________

Staple physician's or other healthcare provider's business card or write in contact information here.

Referred by:

____

Diagnosis

Include relevant vital sign measurements as medical personnel complete your evaluation. (Reference key on page xi.)

BP ________ HR________ Tp________ Rp________

HT ________ Wt________ GL ________ Ch ________

Other ______________________________

Actions Needed *(follow-up, referral, prescriptions, tests, etc.)*

Date Scheduled

Outcome

Healthcare Concern/Questions/Symptoms

Date ____________

Staple physician's or other healthcare provider's business card or write in contact information here.

Referred by: ____________________

Include relevant vital sign measurements as medical personnel complete your evaluation. (Reference key on page xi.)

BP ________ HR________ Tp________ Rp________

HT________ Wt________ GL ________ Ch ________

Other ____________________

Diagnosis

Actions Needed *(follow-up, referral, prescriptions, tests, etc.)*

Date Scheduled

Outcome

Personal Healthcare Record for: ______________________________ *Page* ________

Healthcare Concern/Questions/Symptoms

Date ____________

Staple physician's or other healthcare provider's business card or write in contact information here.

Referred by:

Include relevant vital sign measurements as medical personnel complete your evaluation. (Reference key on page xi.)

BP ________ HR________ Tp________ Rp________

HT ________ Wt________ GL ________ Ch ________

Other ______________________________

Diagnosis

Actions Needed *(follow-up, referral, prescriptions, tests, etc.)* Date Scheduled

Outcome

Personal Healthcare Record for: ______________________________ *Page* __________

Healthcare Concern/Questions/Symptoms

Date ____________

Staple physician's or other healthcare provider's business card or write in contact information here.

Referred by:

____

Include relevant vital sign measurements as medical personnel complete your evaluation. (Reference key on page xi.)

BP ________ HR________ Tp________ Rp________

HT________ Wt________ GL ________ Ch ________

Other ______________________________

Diagnosis

Actions Needed *(follow-up, referral, prescriptions, tests, etc.)* Date Scheduled

Outcome

Healthcare Concern/Questions/Symptoms

Date ____________

Staple physician's or other healthcare provider's business card or write in contact information here.

Referred by:

____

Include relevant vital sign measurements as medical personnel complete your evaluation. (Reference key on page xi.)

BP ________ HR________ Tp________ Rp________

HT ________ Wt________ GL ________ Ch ________

Other ______________________________

Diagnosis

Actions Needed *(follow-up, referral, prescriptions, tests, etc.)* Date Scheduled

Outcome

Healthcare Concern/Questions/Symptoms

Date ____________

Staple physician's or other healthcare provider's business card or write in contact information here.

Referred by:

____

Diagnosis

Include relevant vital sign measurements as medical personnel complete your evaluation. (Reference key on page xi.)

BP ________ HR________ Tp________ Rp________

HT________ Wt________ GL________ Ch________

Other ______________________________

Actions Needed *(follow-up, referral, prescriptions, tests, etc.)*

Date Scheduled

Outcome

Personal Healthcare Record for: ______________________________ *Page* ________

Date ____________

Healthcare Concern/Questions/Symptoms

Staple physician's or other healthcare provider's business card or write in contact information here.

Referred by:

Include relevant vital sign measurements as medical personnel complete your evaluation. (Reference key on page xi.)

BP ________ HR________ Tp________ Rp________

HT________ Wt________ GL ________ Ch ________

Other ______________________________

Diagnosis

Actions Needed *(follow-up, referral, prescriptions, tests, etc.)* Date Scheduled

Outcome

Healthcare Concern/Questions/Symptoms

Date ____________

Staple physician's or other healthcare provider's business card or write in contact information here.

Referred by:

____

Diagnosis

Include relevant vital sign measurements as medical personnel complete your evaluation. (Reference key on page xi.)

BP ________ HR________ Tp________ Rp________

HT________ Wt________ GL ________ Ch ________

Other ______________________________

Actions Needed *(follow-up, referral, prescriptions, tests, etc.)*

Date Scheduled

Outcome

Date ______________

Healthcare Concern/Questions/Symptoms

Staple physician's or other healthcare provider's business card or write in contact information here.

Referred by:

____

Include relevant vital sign measurements as medical personnel complete your evaluation. (Reference key on page xi.)

BP ________ HR________ Tp________ Rp________

HT ________ Wt________ GL ________ Ch ________

Other ______________________________

Diagnosis

Actions Needed *(follow-up, referral, prescriptions, tests, etc.)* Date Scheduled

Outcome

Date ____________

Healthcare Concern/Questions/Symptoms

Staple physician's or other healthcare provider's business card or write in contact information here.

Referred by:

____

Include relevant vital sign measurements as medical personnel complete your evaluation. (Reference key on page xi.)

BP ________ HR________ Tp________ Rp________

HT________ Wt________ GL________ Ch________

Other ______________________________

Diagnosis

Actions Needed *(follow-up, referral, prescriptions, tests, etc.)*

Date Scheduled

Outcome

Healthcare Concern/Questions/Symptoms

Date ____________

Staple physician's or other healthcare provider's business card or write in contact information here.

Referred by:

____

Include relevant vital sign measurements as medical personnel complete your evaluation. (Reference key on page xi.)

BP ________ HR________ Tp________ Rp________

HT ________ Wt________ GL ________ Ch ________

Other ______________________________

Diagnosis

Actions Needed *(follow-up, referral, prescriptions, tests, etc.)* Date Scheduled

Outcome

Healthcare Concern/Questions/Symptoms

Date ________

Staple physician's or other healthcare provider's business card or write in contact information here.

Referred by:

____

Include relevant vital sign measurements as medical personnel complete your evaluation. (Reference key on page xi.)

BP ________ HR________ Tp________ Rp________

HT________ Wt________ GL ________ Ch ________

Other ________________

Diagnosis

Actions Needed *(follow-up, referral, prescriptions, tests, etc.)*

Date Scheduled

Outcome

Date ________

Healthcare Concern/Questions/Symptoms

Staple physician's or other healthcare provider's business card or write in contact information here.

Referred by:

____

Include relevant vital sign measurements as medical personnel complete your evaluation. (Reference key on page xi.)

BP ________ HR________ Tp________ Rp________

HT ________ Wt________ GL ________ Ch ________

Other ________________________

Diagnosis

Actions Needed *(follow-up, referral, prescriptions, tests, etc.)* Date Scheduled

Outcome

Personal Healthcare Record for: ______________________________ *Page* ________

Healthcare Concern/Questions/Symptoms

Date ____________

Staple physician's or other healthcare provider's business card or write in contact information here.

Referred by:

____

Include relevant vital sign measurements as medical personnel complete your evaluation. (Reference key on page xi.)

BP ________ HR________ Tp________ Rp________

HT________ Wt________ GL________ Ch________

Other ______________________________

Diagnosis

Actions Needed *(follow-up, referral, prescriptions, tests, etc.)*

Date Scheduled

Outcome

Healthcare Concern/Questions/Symptoms

Date ____________

Staple physician's or other healthcare provider's business card or write in contact information here.

Referred by:

____

Include relevant vital sign measurements as medical personnel complete your evaluation. (Reference key on page xi.)

BP ________ HR________ Tp________ Rp________

HT________ Wt________ GL ________ Ch ________

Other ______________________________

Diagnosis

Actions Needed *(follow-up, referral, prescriptions, tests, etc.)* Date Scheduled

Outcome

Healthcare Concern/Questions/Symptoms

Date ____________

Staple physician's or other healthcare provider's business card or write in contact information here.

Referred by: ____________________

Diagnosis

Include relevant vital sign measurements as medical personnel complete your evaluation. (Reference key on page xi.)

BP ________ HR________ Tp________ Rp________

HT________ Wt________ GL ________ Ch ________

Other ____________________

Actions Needed *(follow-up, referral, prescriptions, tests, etc.)* Date Scheduled

Outcome

Healthcare Concern/Questions/Symptoms

Date ____________

Staple physician's or other healthcare provider's business card or write in contact information here.

Referred by:

____

Include relevant vital sign measurements as medical personnel complete your evaluation. (Reference key on page xi.)

BP ________ HR________ Tp________ Rp________

HT ________ Wt________ GL ________ Ch ________

Other ______________________________

Diagnosis

Actions Needed *(follow-up, referral, prescriptions, tests, etc.)*

Date Scheduled

Outcome

Healthcare Concern/Questions/Symptoms

Date ________

Staple physician's or other healthcare provider's business card or write in contact information here.

Referred by:

____

Include relevant vital sign measurements as medical personnel complete your evaluation. (Reference key on page xi.)

BP ________ HR________ Tp________ Rp________

HT________ Wt________ GL ________ Ch ________

Other ______________________

Diagnosis

Actions Needed *(follow-up, referral, prescriptions, tests, etc.)*

Date Scheduled

Outcome

Healthcare Concern/Questions/Symptoms

Date ____________

Staple physician's or other healthcare provider's business card or write in contact information here.

Referred by:

____

Diagnosis

Include relevant vital sign measurements as medical personnel complete your evaluation. (Reference key on page xi.)

BP ________ HR________ Tp________ Rp________

HT ________ Wt________ GL ________ Ch ________

Other ______________________

Actions Needed *(follow-up, referral, prescriptions, tests, etc.)*

Date Scheduled

Outcome

Personal Healthcare Record for: ______________________________ *Page* __________

Healthcare Concern/Questions/Symptoms

Date ____________

Staple physician's or other healthcare provider's business card or write in contact information here.

Referred by:

____

Include relevant vital sign measurements as medical personnel complete your evaluation. (Reference key on page xi.)

BP ________ HR________ Tp________ Rp________

HT________ Wt________ GL________ Ch________

Other ______________________________

Diagnosis

Actions Needed *(follow-up, referral, prescriptions, tests, etc.)* Date Scheduled

Outcome

Healthcare Concern/Questions/Symptoms

Date ____________

Staple physician's or other healthcare provider's business card or write in contact information here.

Referred by:

____

Include relevant vital sign measurements as medical personnel complete your evaluation. (Reference key on page xi.)

BP ______ HR______ Tp______ Rp______

HT______ Wt______ GL ______ Ch ______

Other ______________________

Diagnosis

Actions Needed *(follow-up, referral, prescriptions, tests, etc.)*

Date Scheduled

Outcome

Personal Healthcare Record for: ______________________________ *Page* ________

Healthcare Concern/Questions/Symptoms

Date ____________

Staple physician's or other healthcare provider's business card or write in contact information here.

Referred by:

____

Include relevant vital sign measurements as medical personnel complete your evaluation. (Reference key on page xi.)

BP ________ HR________ Tp________ Rp________

HT________ Wt________ GL ________ Ch________

Other ______________________________

Diagnosis

Actions Needed *(follow-up, referral, prescriptions, tests, etc.)* Date Scheduled

Outcome

Healthcare Concern/Questions/Symptoms

Date ______________

Staple physician's or other healthcare provider's business card or write in contact information here.

Referred by:

____

Include relevant vital sign measurements as medical personnel complete your evaluation. (Reference key on page xi.)

BP ________ HR________ Tp________ Rp________

HT ________ Wt________ GL ________ Ch ________

Other ______________________________

Diagnosis

Actions Needed *(follow-up, referral, prescriptions, tests, etc.)*

Date Scheduled

Outcome

Personal Healthcare Record for: ____________________ *Page* ________

Date ____________

Healthcare Concern/Questions/Symptoms

Staple physician's or other healthcare provider's business card or write in contact information here.

Referred by:

____

Include relevant vital sign measurements as medical personnel complete your evaluation. (Reference key on page xi.)

BP ________ HR________ Tp________ Rp________

HT________ Wt________ GL________ Ch_______

Other ____________________

Diagnosis

Actions Needed *(follow-up, referral, prescriptions, tests, etc.)* Date Scheduled

Outcome

Healthcare Concern/Questions/Symptoms

Date ____________

Staple physician's or other healthcare provider's business card or write in contact information here.

Referred by:

____

Diagnosis

Include relevant vital sign measurements as medical personnel complete your evaluation. (Reference key on page xi.)

BP ________ HR________ Tp________ Rp________

HT________ Wt________ GL________ Ch_______

Other ______________________________

Actions Needed *(follow-up, referral, prescriptions, tests, etc.)*

Date Scheduled

Outcome

Date ____________

Healthcare Concern/Questions/Symptoms

Staple physician's or other healthcare provider's business card or write in contact information here.

Referred by:

____

Include relevant vital sign measurements as medical personnel complete your evaluation. (Reference key on page xi.)

BP ______ HR______ Tp______ Rp______

HT______ Wt______ GL______ Ch______

Other ____________________

Diagnosis

Actions Needed *(follow-up, referral, prescriptions, tests, etc.)* Date Scheduled

Outcome

Healthcare Concern/Questions/Symptoms

Date ____________

____

____

____

____

____

____

____

____

Staple physician's or other healthcare provider's business card or write in contact information here.

Referred by:

____

Include relevant vital sign measurements as medical personnel complete your evaluation. (Reference key on page xi.)

BP ________ HR________ Tp________ Rp________

HT________ Wt________ GL ________ Ch ________

Other ______________________________

____

Diagnosis

____

____

____

____

____

____

Actions Needed *(follow-up, referral, prescriptions, tests, etc.)* Date Scheduled

____

____

____

____

Outcome

____

____

____

____

Date ____________

Healthcare Concern/Questions/Symptoms

Staple physician's or other healthcare provider's business card or write in contact information here.

Referred by:

____

Diagnosis

Include relevant vital sign measurements as medical personnel complete your evaluation. (Reference key on page xi.)

BP ________ HR________ Tp________ Rp________

HT________ Wt________ GL ________ Ch _______

Other ______________________________

Actions Needed *(follow-up, referral, prescriptions, tests, etc.)* Date Scheduled

Outcome

Date ______________

Healthcare Concern/Questions/Symptoms

____

____

____

____

____

____

____

____

Include relevant vital sign measurements as medical personnel complete your evaluation. (Reference key on page xi.)

BP ________ HR________ Tp________ Rp________

HT________ Wt________ GL________ Ch________

Other ______________________________

____

Staple physician's or other healthcare provider's business card or write in contact information here.

Referred by:

____

Diagnosis

____

____

____

____

____

____

Actions Needed *(follow-up, referral, prescriptions, tests, etc.)* Date Scheduled

____

____

____

____

Outcome

____

____

____

____

Date ______________

Healthcare Concern/Questions/Symptoms

Staple physician's or other healthcare provider's business card or write in contact information here.

Referred by:

____

Diagnosis

Include relevant vital sign measurements as medical personnel complete your evaluation. (Reference key on page xi.)

BP ________ HR________ Tp________ Rp________

HT________ Wt________ GL ________ Ch_______

Other ______________________

Actions Needed *(follow-up, referral, prescriptions, tests, etc.)*

Date Scheduled

Outcome

Personal Healthcare Record for: ______________________________ *Page* __________

Healthcare Concern/Questions/Symptoms

Date ______________

Staple physician's or other healthcare provider's business card or write in contact information here.

Referred by:

____

Diagnosis

Include relevant vital sign measurements as medical personnel complete your evaluation. (Reference key on page xi.)

BP ________ HR________ Tp________ Rp________

HT ________ Wt________ GL ________ Ch _______

Other ______________________________

Actions Needed *(follow-up, referral, prescriptions, tests, etc.)* Date Scheduled

Outcome

Healthcare Concern/Questions/Symptoms

Date ______________

Staple physician's or other healthcare provider's business card or write in contact information here.

Referred by:

____

Diagnosis

Include relevant vital sign measurements as medical personnel complete your evaluation. (Reference key on page xi.)

BP ________ HR________ Tp________ Rp________

HT________ Wt________ GL ________ Ch________

Other ______________________________

Actions Needed *(follow-up, referral, prescriptions, tests, etc.)*

Date Scheduled

Outcome

Date ________

Healthcare Concern/Questions/Symptoms

Staple physician's or other healthcare provider's business card or write in contact information here.

Referred by:

Include relevant vital sign measurements as medical personnel complete your evaluation. (Reference key on page xi.)

BP ______ HR______ Tp______ Rp______

HT______ Wt______ GL ______ Ch ______

Other ________________

Diagnosis

Actions Needed *(follow-up, referral, prescriptions, tests, etc.)* Date Scheduled

Outcome

Healthcare Concern/Questions/Symptoms

Date ________

Staple physician's or other healthcare provider's business card or write in contact information here.

Referred by:

____

Include relevant vital sign measurements as medical personnel complete your evaluation. (Reference key on page xi.)

BP ________ HR________ Tp________ Rp________

HT________ Wt________ GL ________ Ch ________

Other ______________________________

Diagnosis

Actions Needed *(follow-up, referral, prescriptions, tests, etc.)*

Date Scheduled

Outcome

Date ______________

Healthcare Concern/Questions/Symptoms

Staple physician's or other healthcare provider's business card or write in contact information here.

Referred by:

____

Include relevant vital sign measurements as medical personnel complete your evaluation. (Reference key on page xi.)

BP ________ HR________ Tp________ Rp________

HT________ Wt________ GL________ Ch________

Other ______________________________

Diagnosis

Actions Needed *(follow-up, referral, prescriptions, tests, etc.)* Date Scheduled

Outcome

Date ____________

Healthcare Concern/Questions/Symptoms

Include relevant vital sign measurements as medical personnel complete your evaluation. (Reference key on page xi.)

BP ______ HR______ Tp______ Rp______

HT______ Wt______ GL ______ Ch______

Other ______________________________

Staple physician's or other healthcare provider's business card or write in contact information here.

Referred by:

____

Diagnosis

Actions Needed *(follow-up, referral, prescriptions, tests, etc.)* Date Scheduled

Outcome

Personal Healthcare Record for: ______________________ *Page* ________

Date ________

Healthcare Concern/Questions/Symptoms

Staple physician's or other healthcare provider's business card or write in contact information here.

Referred by:

____

Include relevant vital sign measurements as medical personnel complete your evaluation. (Reference key on page xi.)

BP ________ HR________ Tp________ Rp________

HT________ Wt________ GL________ Ch________

Other ______________________

Diagnosis

Actions Needed *(follow-up, referral, prescriptions, tests, etc.)*

Date Scheduled

Outcome

Healthcare Concern/Questions/Symptoms

Date ________

Staple physician's or other healthcare provider's business card or write in contact information here.

Referred by:

____

Include relevant vital sign measurements as medical personnel complete your evaluation. (Reference key on page xi.)

BP ______ HR______ Tp______ Rp______

HT______ Wt______ GL ______ Ch______

Other ________________

Diagnosis

Actions Needed *(follow-up, referral, prescriptions, tests, etc.)* Date Scheduled

Outcome

Healthcare Concern/Questions/Symptoms

Date ______

Staple physician's or other healthcare provider's business card or write in contact information here.

Referred by: ______

Diagnosis

Include relevant vital sign measurements as medical personnel complete your evaluation. (Reference key on page xi.)

BP ______ HR______ Tp______ Rp______

HT______ Wt______ GL ______ Ch ______

Other ______

Actions Needed *(follow-up, referral, prescriptions, tests, etc.)* Date Scheduled

Outcome

Date ____________

Healthcare Concern/Questions/Symptoms

Staple physician's or other healthcare provider's business card or write in contact information here.

Referred by:

Include relevant vital sign measurements as medical personnel complete your evaluation. (Reference key on page xi.)

BP ________ HR________ Tp________ Rp________

HT________ Wt________ GL ________ Ch ________

Other ______________________________

Diagnosis

Actions Needed *(follow-up, referral, prescriptions, tests, etc.)*

Date Scheduled

Outcome

Healthcare Concern/Questions/Symptoms

Date ____________

Staple physician's or other healthcare provider's business card or write in contact information here.

Referred by:

____

Include relevant vital sign measurements as medical personnel complete your evaluation. (Reference key on page xi.)

BP ________ HR________ Tp________ Rp________

HT________ Wt________ GL ________ Ch ________

Other ______________________

Diagnosis

Actions Needed *(follow-up, referral, prescriptions, tests, etc.)*

Date Scheduled

Outcome

Healthcare Concern/Questions/Symptoms

Date ____________

Staple physician's or other healthcare provider's business card or write in contact information here.

Referred by:

____

Include relevant vital sign measurements as medical personnel complete your evaluation. (Reference key on page xi.)

BP ________ HR________ Tp________ Rp________

HT________ Wt________ GL________ Ch________

Other ______________________

Diagnosis

Actions Needed *(follow-up, referral, prescriptions, tests, etc.)*

Date Scheduled

Outcome

Date ______

Healthcare Concern/Questions/Symptoms

Staple physician's or other healthcare provider's business card or write in contact information here.

Referred by:

Include relevant vital sign measurements as medical personnel complete your evaluation. (Reference key on page xi.)

BP ______ HR______ Tp______ Rp______

HT______ Wt______ GL ______ Ch ______

Other ______

Diagnosis

Actions Needed *(follow-up, referral, prescriptions, tests, etc.)* Date Scheduled

Outcome

Personal Healthcare Record for: ______________________________ *Page* ________

Healthcare Concern/Questions/Symptoms

Date ____________

Staple physician's or other healthcare provider's business card or write in contact information here.

Referred by:

____

Include relevant vital sign measurements as medical personnel complete your evaluation. (Reference key on page xi.)

BP ________ HR________ Tp________ Rp________

HT________ Wt________ GL ________ Ch ________

Other ______________________________

Diagnosis

Actions Needed *(follow-up, referral, prescriptions, tests, etc.)*

Date Scheduled

Outcome

Healthcare Concern/Questions/Symptoms

Date ____________

Staple physician's or other healthcare provider's business card or write in contact information here.

Referred by:

____

Include relevant vital sign measurements as medical personnel complete your evaluation. (Reference key on page xi.)

BP ________ HR________ Tp________ Rp________

HT________ Wt________ GL ________ Ch________

Other ______________________

Diagnosis

Actions Needed *(follow-up, referral, prescriptions, tests, etc.)*

Date Scheduled

Outcome

Healthcare Concern/Questions/Symptoms

Date ____________

Staple physician's or other healthcare provider's business card or write in contact information here.

Referred by:

____

Include relevant vital sign measurements as medical personnel complete your evaluation. (Reference key on page xi.)

BP ________ HR________ Tp________ Rp________

HT________ Wt________ GL ________ Ch_______

Other ____________________

Diagnosis

Actions Needed *(follow-up, referral, prescriptions, tests, etc.)* Date Scheduled

Outcome

Personal Healthcare Record for: ______________________________ *Page* __________

Healthcare Concern/Questions/Symptoms

Date ______________

Staple physician's or other healthcare provider's business card or write in contact information here.

Referred by:

____

Include relevant vital sign measurements as medical personnel complete your evaluation. (Reference key on page xi.)

BP ________ HR________ Tp________ Rp________

HT________ Wt________ GL ________ Ch ________

Other ______________________________

Diagnosis

Actions Needed *(follow-up, referral, prescriptions, tests, etc.)* Date Scheduled

Outcome

Healthcare Concern/Questions/Symptoms

Date ______

Staple physician's or other healthcare provider's business card or write in contact information here.

Referred by:

____

Include relevant vital sign measurements as medical personnel complete your evaluation. (Reference key on page xi.)

BP ______ HR______ Tp______ Rp______

HT______ Wt______ GL ______ Ch ______

Other ______________________

Diagnosis

Actions Needed *(follow-up, referral, prescriptions, tests, etc.)*

Date Scheduled

Outcome

Date ____________

Healthcare Concern/Questions/Symptoms

Staple physician's or other healthcare provider's business card or write in contact information here.

Referred by:

____

Include relevant vital sign measurements as medical personnel complete your evaluation. (Reference key on page xi.)

BP ______ HR______ Tp______ Rp______

HT______ Wt______ GL ______ Ch______

Other ________________________

Diagnosis

Actions Needed *(follow-up, referral, prescriptions, tests, etc.)* Date Scheduled

Outcome

Date ____________

Healthcare Concern/Questions/Symptoms

Staple physician's or other healthcare provider's business card or write in contact information here.

Referred by:

____

Include relevant vital sign measurements as medical personnel complete your evaluation. (Reference key on page xi.)

BP ______ HR______ Tp______ Rp______

HT______ Wt______ GL______ Ch______

Other ______________________

Diagnosis

Actions Needed *(follow-up, referral, prescriptions, tests, etc.)* Date Scheduled

Outcome

Personal Healthcare Record for: ______________________________ *Page* ________

Healthcare Concern/Questions/Symptoms

Date ____________

Staple physician's or other healthcare provider's business card or write in contact information here.

Referred by:

____

Include relevant vital sign measurements as medical personnel complete your evaluation. (Reference key on page xi.)

BP ________ HR________ Tp________ Rp________

HT________ Wt________ GL________ Ch________

Other ______________________________

Diagnosis

Actions Needed *(follow-up, referral, prescriptions, tests, etc.)* Date Scheduled

Outcome

Personal Healthcare Record for: ______________________________ *Page* ________

Healthcare Concern/Questions/Symptoms

Date ____________

Staple physician's or other healthcare provider's business card or write in contact information here.

Referred by:

____

Diagnosis

Include relevant vital sign measurements as medical personnel complete your evaluation. (Reference key on page xi.)

BP ________ HR________ Tp________ Rp________

HT________ Wt________ GL________ Ch________

Other ______________________________

Actions Needed *(follow-up, referral, prescriptions, tests, etc.)*

Date Scheduled

Outcome

Personal Healthcare Record for: ______________________ *Page* ________

Date ________

Healthcare Concern/Questions/Symptoms

Staple physician's or other healthcare provider's business card or write in contact information here.

Referred by: ________________

Diagnosis

Include relevant vital sign measurements as medical personnel complete your evaluation. (Reference key on page xi.)

BP ________ HR________ Tp________ Rp________

HT________ Wt________ GL ________ Ch ________

Other ______________________

Actions Needed *(follow-up, referral, prescriptions, tests, etc.)*

Date Scheduled

Outcome

Healthcare Concern/Questions/Symptoms

Date ____________

Staple physician's or other healthcare provider's business card or write in contact information here.

Referred by:

____

Diagnosis

Include relevant vital sign measurements as medical personnel complete your evaluation. (Reference key on page xi.)

BP ________ HR________ Tp________ Rp________

HT________ Wt________ GL ________ Ch ________

Other ______________________________

Actions Needed *(follow-up, referral, prescriptions, tests, etc.)*

Date Scheduled

Outcome

Healthcare Concern/Questions/Symptoms

Date ____________

Staple physician's or other healthcare provider's business card or write in contact information here.

Referred by:

____

Diagnosis

Include relevant vital sign measurements as medical personnel complete your evaluation. (Reference key on page xi.)

BP ________ HR________ Tp________ Rp________

HT________ Wt________ GL ________ Ch ________

Other ______________________________

Actions Needed *(follow-up, referral, prescriptions, tests, etc.)*

Date Scheduled

Outcome

Healthcare Concern/Questions/Symptoms

Date ____________

Staple physician's or other healthcare provider's business card or write in contact information here.

Referred by:

____

Include relevant vital sign measurements as medical personnel complete your evaluation. (Reference key on page xi.)

BP ______ HR______ Tp______ Rp______

HT______ Wt______ GL ______ Ch ______

Other ______________________

Diagnosis

Actions Needed *(follow-up, referral, prescriptions, tests, etc.)* Date Scheduled

Outcome

Date ________

Healthcare Concern/Questions/Symptoms

Staple physician's or other healthcare provider's business card or write in contact information here.

Referred by:

____

Diagnosis

Include relevant vital sign measurements as medical personnel complete your evaluation. (Reference key on page xi.)

BP ________ HR________ Tp________ Rp________

HT________ Wt________ GL________ Ch________

Other ________

Actions Needed *(follow-up, referral, prescriptions, tests, etc.)* Date Scheduled

Outcome

SECTION B

Health History

Don't Forget

Personal Healthcare Record

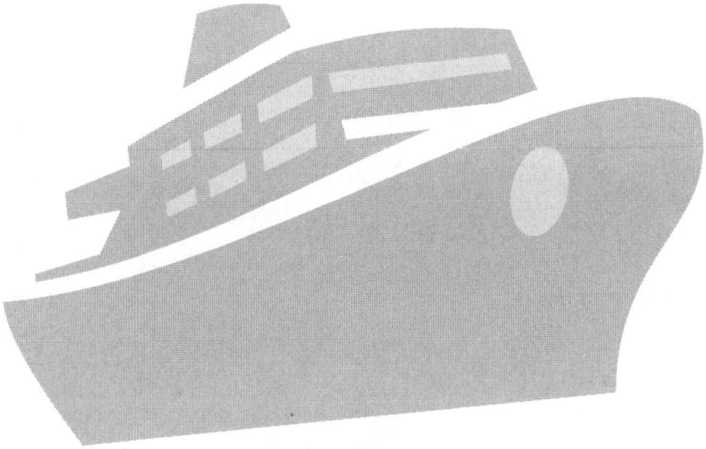

Health History

At-a-Glance

Note: We strongly recommend putting this page in a protector and placing it at the very beginning of the PHR so it may serve as a quick reference for emergency personnel. See pages 75-95 for detailed Health History information.

Your Name ______________________ Home Phone ______________________

Address ____

City, State, Zip ______________________________

Current Photo

Current Medications *include over the counter medications and supplements.* (see page 78)

____

____

Current Critical or Chronic Conditions

Note: If you have any of the conditions on page 79, especially conditions noted in BOLD, note them in this section.

Known Allergies (see page 75)

____

____

Drugs ____

____

Food ____

____

Other ____

Emergency Contact(s)

____

Name/Relationship | Phone – Home | Cell

	Circle		
Health Insurance	No	Yes	*(see page 77)*
Advance Medical Directive	No	Yes	*(see page 95)*
Religious Preference	______________		
Organ donor	No	Yes	
Contact lenses	No	Yes	
Hearing Aids	No	Yes	
Dentures	No	Yes	
Metal Prosthesis or Implants	No	Yes	Location: ______________

____

Primary Care Physician | Phone

Note: Continue on back of this page if more space is needed.
Emergency personnel, please photocopy and return this sheet to patient.

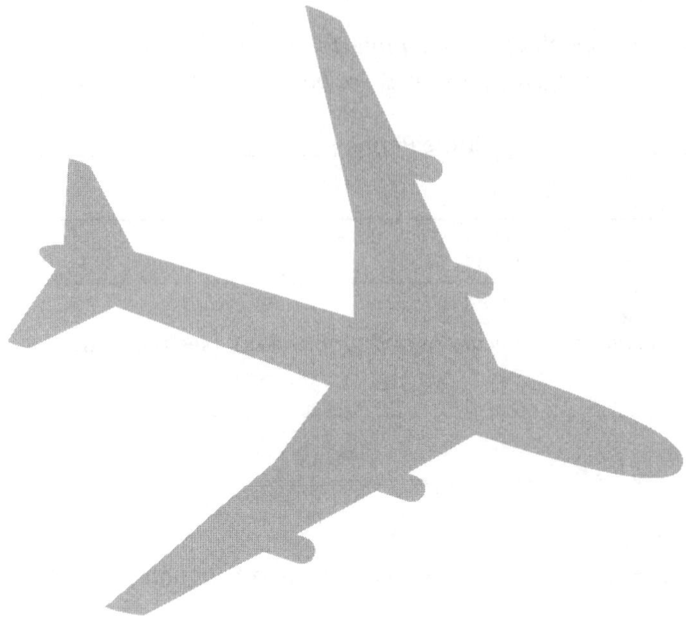

Wallet Card

Complete the wallet card information below and cut out to carry in your wallet for a quick reference. If additional space is needed, make a second card from the template and fold together with the one provided. Review and update information annually or anytime your information changes. Card stock is recommended, but not necessary, for durability.

FRONT

CUT OUT — FOLD HERE — FOLD HERE

MEDICAL INFORMATION

Pharmacy: ____________

Phone: ____________

Surgeries: ____________

____

____

____

Allergies: ____________

____

____

Eye Glass/Contact Perscription:

____

Blood Type: ____________

PHYSICIAN INFORMATION

Physician: ____________

Phone: ____________

Physician: ____________

Phone: ____________

EMERGENCY CONTACT:

Name: ____________

Address: ____________

____

____

Phone: ____________

POCKET REFERENCE

Personal Healthcare Record

Don't Forget

Name ____________

CONFIDENTIAL

If found, please return to Emergency Contact

BACK

MEDICATIONS	DOSAGE	TIMES/ DAY	DATE STARTED	CONDITION

Health History

Personal Information

Note: For convenience, the following information can be photocopied and provided to your healthcare provider. Complete any of the information that could change in pencil. Use ink for permanent information. Include this information on your wallet card, too!

Your Name ______________________ Home Phone ______________________

Address ______________________

City, State, Zip ______________________

Email Address ______________________

Blood Type ______________________

Note: Current Healthcare Provider information is listed on each journal page and on page 76.

Known Allergies

Name of Drug, Food, Plant, Other	Typical Reactions Comments, Treatment	First Developed

Religious Preference: ______________________

Emergency Contact(s)

Name ______________________ Home Phone ______________________

Address ______________________ Cell ______________________

City, State, Zip ______________________

Advance Medical Directive

Note: Place a copy of your Advance Medical Directive at the back of the Medical History section (page 95).

Date Completed ______________________ Location ______________________

Healthcare Provider Contact Information

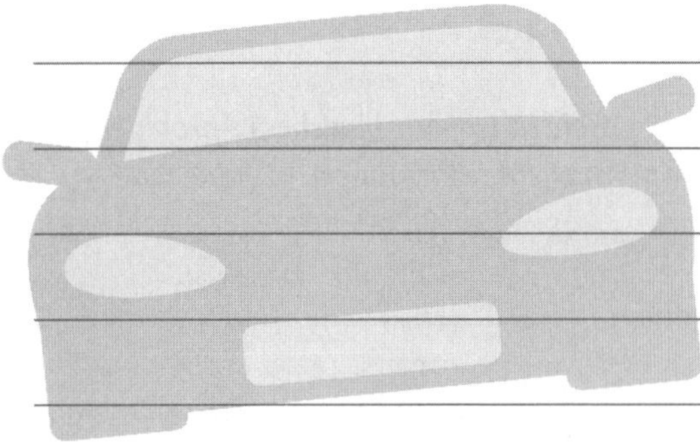

Health Insurance

Hint: Copy the front and back of all current insurance cards and keep these copies in your PHR. We also recommend getting signed Insurance Verification forms from any new healthcare professionals you may visit (see Template/Section page 111).

Primary Insurance Company ______________________

Group/Policy Number ______________ Member ID Number ______________

Address ______________________ Phone ______________

Member Name ______________________

Secondary Insurance Company ______________________

Group/Policy Number ______________ Member ID Number ______________

Address ______________________ Phone ______________

Member Name ______________________

Prescription Drug Service ______________________

Group/Policy Number ______________ Member ID Number ______________

Address ______________________ Phone ______________

Member Name ______________________

Medicare Part B Insurance (Carrier) ______________________

Group/Policy Number ______________ Member ID Number ______________

Address ______________________ Phone ______________

Medicare Part A Insurance (Fiscal Intermediary) ______________________

Group/Policy Number ______________ Member ID Number ______________

Address ______________________ Phone ______________

Medicare Supplemental Insurance ______________________

Group/Policy Number ______________ Member ID Number ______________

Address ______________________ Phone ______________

Other Insurance Information

____

____

____

Medications

Note: Include this information on the wallet card. Include over the counter medications and supplements.

Medications	Dosage	Times/Day	Date Started	Condition

Common Health Conditions

Indicate if you have or have in the past been diagnosed with any of the following by placing a date or approximate date the problem began.

Health Condition	Date Began	Health Condition	Date Began
Acid reflux		Hypertension	
AIDS, AIDS related disorders		Insomnia	
Angina		Kidney disease	
Anxiety		Liver disease	
Aneurysm		Meningitis	
Arrhythmia		Mental/Nervous Disorders	
Arthritis		Migraine	
Asthma		Muscular dystrophy	
Back Pain		Musculoskeletal/joint problems	
Bipolar disorder		Myocardial infarction	
Bleeding or blood disorder		Nasal polyps	
Blood clots and VTE		Nausea, gas, indigestion	
Bronchitis		Pancreas	
Cancer		Peptic ulcer	
Chest pain		Rectal problems	
Chronic obstructive pulmonary disease (COPD)		Rhinitis	
Constipation, loose bowels, diarrhea		Rheumatic fever	
Cystic fibrosis		Shortness of breath	
Depression		Sinusitis	
Diabetes		Sleeping problems	
Dizziness		Stomach problems	
Endocrine problems		Tired, unusually	
Epilepsy		Tuberculosis	
Fainting spells		Tumor	
Gall bladder		Other – list below	
Gastroesophageal reflux disease (GERD/ GORD)			
Hay fever			
Headaches			
Heart attack			
Heart failure			
Heart murmur			
Heartburn			
Hernia			
High blood pressure			
High cholesterol			

Early Childhood

Birth

Date ________________ Time ________________

Weight ____________ Length ____________ Hair Color ____________ Eye Color ____________

Location ______________________________ Doctor ________________

Address ____

Condition of health at birth: (circle one) Normal Complications

Complications? Please describe. ________________________________

Vaccinations and Immunizations

Shots/Other Procedures	Site on Body	Reactions/Results	Action

Update for Biological Parent and Sibling Health Summary

Health of Parents, Siblings, Blood Relatives

Hint: Note Date Updated *(Recommend annually or if any major changes occur.)* ______________________

____

Biological Mother: Date of birth ________________ Name ______________________________

If living, condition of health : excellent good fair poor Male Female

Why? ____

____

____

____

Major health concerns: ____

____

____

____

If deceased, age ________ Cause of death ______________________________________

Biological Father: Date of birth ________________ Name ______________________________

If living, condition of health : excellent good fair poor

Why? ____

____

____

____

Major health concerns: ____

____

____

____

If deceased, age ________ Cause of death ______________________________________

Hint: If needed, before completing this page, make additional pages for additional family members.

Biological Sibling: Date of birth ____________________ Name ____

If living, condition of health : excellent good fair poor Male Female

Why? ____

____

Major health concerns: ____

____

If deceased, age __________ Cause of death ____

Biological Sibling: Date of birth ____________________ Name ____

If living, condition of health : excellent good fair poor Male Female

Why? ____

____

Major health concerns: ____

____

If deceased, age __________ Cause of death ____

Biological Sibling: Date of birth ____________________ Name ____

If living, condition of health : excellent good fair poor Male Female

Why? ____

____

Major health concerns: ____

____

If deceased, age __________ Cause of death ____

Biological Mother's Side

Hint: If needed, before completing this page, make additional pages for additional family members.

(Other blood relatives who have/had critical medical conditions grandparents, aunts, uncles.)

Relationship ____________ Name ____________

Date of birth ____________

If living, condition of health : excellent good fair poor Male Female

Why? ____________

____

Major health concerns: ____________

____

If deceased, age ______ Cause of death ____________

Relationship ____________ Name ____________

Date of birth ____________

If living, condition of health : excellent good fair poor Male Female

Why? ____________

____

Major health concerns: ____________

____

If deceased, age ______ Cause of death ____________

Relationship ____________ Name ____________

Date of birth ____________

If living, condition of health : excellent good fair poor Male Female

Why? ____________

____

Major health concerns: ____________

____

If deceased, age ______ Cause of death ____________

Biological Father's Side

Hint: If needed, before completing this page, make additional pages for additional family members.

(Other blood relatives who have/had critical medical conditions grandparents, aunts, uncles.)

Relationship ____________________ Name ____

Date of birth ____________________

If living, condition of health : excellent good fair poor Male Female

Why? ____

____

Major health concerns: ____

____

If deceased, age ________ Cause of death ____

Relationship ____________________ Name ____

Date of birth ____________________

If living, condition of health : excellent good fair poor Male Female

Why? ____

____

Major health concerns: ____

____

If deceased, age ________ Cause of death ____

Relationship ____________________ Name ____

Date of birth ____________________

If living, condition of health : excellent good fair poor Male Female

Why? ____

____

Major health concerns: ____

____

If deceased, age ________ Cause of death ____

Surgeries or Hospitalizations

(Serious Illness or Injury)

Note: See Page 79 for a list of common diseases. Women: include pregnancy information here.

Date	Illness or Injury

Vaccinations and Immunizations

Hint: Not all vaccinations are indicated for all adults. Consult your physician for direction. For additional information contact the Centers for Disease Control and Prevention http://www.cdc.gov

Adult

Vaccine	Defined	Date Given	Type of Vaccine	Site on Body/ Reactions	Doctor's Office or Clinic	Date Next Dose Due
	OPV – oral polio virus IPV – injectable polio virus					
Polio 1						
Polio 2						
Polio 3						
Polio 4						
DTP, Td, DT 1	diphtheria, tetanus, acellular pertussis DTap, Tdap					
DTP, Td, DT 2						
DTP, Td, DT 3						
DTP, Td, DT 4						
DTP, Td, DT 5						
Rota	Rotavirus Gastroenteritis - diarrhea					

Adult, continued

Vaccine	Defined	Date Given	Type of Vaccine	Site on Body/ Reactions	Doctor's Office or Clinic	Date Next Dose Due
MMR 1	mumps, measles, rubella					
MMR 2						
Varicella	chicken pox					
Hib	homophilus influenza type B					
MCV4	meningococcal men-ingitis					
Hep A	hepatitis type A virus					
Hep B 1	hepatitis type B virus					
Hep B 2						
Hep B 3						
TB Skin Test 1	tuberculosis					
TB Skin Test 1						
PCV	ear infections, menin-gitis, pneumonia, and septicemia					
HPV	human papilloma virus					
Influenza Vaccine	flu (annual)					
Zoster	shingles					

Hospitalizations

(Other)

Note: Include this information on the wallet card.

Date	Reason for Hospitalization

Dental Records

(Optional quick cross reference for Journal pages)

Date	Purpose of Visit

Hearing Records

(Optional quick cross reference for Journal pages)

Date	Purpose of Visit	Results

Vision Records

(Optional quick cross reference for Journal pages)

Date	Purpose of Visit	Results Without Correction/With Correction

Development and Identification Photographs

attach photo here

Date: ____________
Age: ____________
Ht: ____________
Wt: ____________

attach photo here

Date: ____________
Age: ____________
Ht: ____________
Wt: ____________

attach photo here

Date: ____________
Age: ____________
Ht: ____________
Wt: ____________

attach photo here

Date: ____________
Age: ____________
Ht: ____________
Wt: ____________

attach photo here

Date: ____________
Age: ____________
Ht: ____________
Wt: ____________

attach photo here

Date: ____________
Age: ____________
Ht: ____________
Wt: ____________

attach photo here

Date: ____________
Age: ____________
Ht: ____________
Wt: ____________

attach photo here

Date: ____________
Age: ____________
Ht: ____________
Wt: ____________

attach photo here

Date: ____________
Age: ____________
Ht: ____________
Wt: ____________

attach photo here

Date: ____________
Age: ____________
Ht: ____________
Wt: ____________

attach photo here

Date: ____________
Age: ____________
Ht: ____________
Wt: ____________

attach photo here

Date: ____________
Age: ____________
Ht: ____________
Wt: ____________

Identification Records

Note: Attach finger print records to this page. Finger printing can be obtained from a variety of locations. Check with your local law enforcement agency.

Note: Insert hair clippings in a small plastic baggie and attach to this page for use in DNA tests, if needed.

Note: Amber Alert GPS for Dementia patients. For more information check www.amberalertgps.com

List device information here.

Advanced Medical Directive

Insert a signed copy of your Advanced Directive here.

Note: For assistance in locating Advance Directive form, contact your local hospital or www.eldercare.gov

SECTION C

Healthcare Reference Information

A section where you can add additional healthcare articles and information, specific to your needs.

Don't Forget

The contents of the Personal Healthcare Record are not designed to offer medical advice or replace your doctor's healthcare advice or records.

Adult Reminders and Checklist

✓	Age	Female	Male
	18-39	• Check height and weight-track changes • Check blood pressure, cholesterol levels, blood sugar levels (signs of diabetes) • Re-immunize, as needed, for tetanus, flu or other concerns your doctor recommends • Check breasts for lumps or other changes • Get a pelvic exam and Pap test as suggested by your doctor • Discuss any other personal concerns you may have (keep notes on your Journal page) • Skin (mole) exam • Thyroid test	• Check height and weight-track changes • Check blood pressure, cholesterol levels, blood sugar levels (signs of diabetes) • Re-immunize, as needed, for tetanus, flu or other concerns your doctor recommends • Check testicles for lumps or other changes • Discuss any other personal concerns you may have (keep notes on your Journal page) • Skin (mole) exam • Thyroid test
	40-64	• Check height and weight-track changes • Check blood pressure, cholesterol, blood sugar levels (signs of diabetes) based on doctor's direction • Check all vital organs for problems • Check breasts for lumps or other changes • Get a pelvic exam and Pap test as suggested by your doctor • Schedule mammogram • Re-immunize, as needed, for tetanus, flu or other concerns your doctor recommends • Discuss getting a colonoscopy (check for colon cancer) Check entire body for suspicious skin changes	• Check height and weight-track changes • Check blood pressure, cholesterol, blood sugar levels (signs of diabetes) based on doctor's direction • Check all vital organs for problems • Re-immunize, as needed, for tetanus, flu or other concerns your doctor recommends • Discuss getting a colonoscopy (check for colon cancer) • Check entire body for suspicious skin changes • Prostate exam and PSA test
	65+	• Check height and weight-track changes • Check blood pressure, cholesterol, blood sugar levels (signs of diabetes) based on doctor's direction • Check all vital organs for problems • Check breasts for lumps or other changes • Get a pelvic exam and Pap test as suggested by your doctor • Schedule mammogram • Re-immunize, as needed, for tetanus, flu or other concerns your doctor recommends • Repeat colonoscopy (check for colon cancer) as directed by your doctor • Check entire body for suspicious skin changes • Get a bone density scan	• Check height and weight-track changes • Check blood pressure, cholesterol, blood sugar levels (signs of diabetes) based on doctor's direction • Check all vital organs for problems • Re-immunize, as needed, for tetanus, flu or other concerns your doctor recommends • Repeat colonoscopy (check for colon cancer) as directed by your doctor • Check entire body for suspicious skin changes • Get a bone density scan

General Range Chart for Common Health Indicators

Individual health conditions vary. The general information provided below, obtained from a variety of public sources, may change due to continued research. The websites listed on page 103 may be consulted for more detailed and up-to-date information.

Caution: The contents of the Personal Healthcare Record are not designed to offer medical advice or replace your doctor's healthcare advice or records.

	Normal/Average Range		
Temperature	97.8 – 99.1 degrees Fahrenheit / average 98.6 degrees Fahrenheit		
Breathing	12-18 breaths per minute		
Blood Pressure	**Adults** *mm of mercury (mm Hg)*	**Systolic** *(top number)*	**Diastolic** *(bottom number)*
	Normal	Less than 120	And Less than 80
	Prehypertension	120–139	Or 80–89
	High Blood Pressure		
	Stage 1	140–159	Or 90–99
	Stage 2	160 or higher	Or 100 or higher

		Beats per minute (resting)
Pulse/Heart Rate	Newborn Infants	100 - 160
	Children 1 – 10 years	70 -100
	Over 10 Years *(includes adults and seniors)*	60 – 100
	Well-trained Athletes	40 – 60
	Exercise Heart Rate	Exercise 60-90% of your maximum heart rate. To determine you maximum heart rate. Subtract your age from 220 to get your beats per minute. Multiply your beats per minute by 0.6 and again by 0.9 to get your personal range.

General Range Chart for Common Health Indicators, continued

Indicator	Category	mg/dL
LDL (Bad) Cholesterol	Optimal	Less than 100
	Near Optimal/ Above Optimal	100 - 129
	Borderline High	130 - 159
	High	160 - 189
	Very High	190 and above

Indicator	Category	Average range in mg/dL *(higher the better)*
HDL (Good) Cholesterol	Men	40 – 50
	Women	50 – 60

Indicator	Category	mg/dL
Triglyceride Level	Normal	Less than 150
	Borderline High	150 - 199
	High	200 - 499
	Very High	500

Indicator	Target Blood Glucose Levels for people with Diabetes	
Blood Glucose	Before meals	70 - 130
	1 – 2 hours after start of meal	less than 180
	Low Blood Glucose (Hypoglycemia)	below 70

Indicator	Body Mass Index (BMI)	
Weight	Healthy	18.5 – 24.9
	Overweight	25 – 29.9
	Obese	30 or greater
	Or consult standard height/weight charts	

Personal Healthcare Record for: " Journal Page Sample " *Page* 10

Healthcare Concern/Questions/Symptoms

Date 1/5/XX

Re-occurring headache

Staple physician's or other healthcare provider's business card or write in contact information here.

Dr. John Doe
123 Any Pl.
Anytown, State 12345
123-456-7890

Referred by: ______

Include relevant measurements as medical personnel complete your evaluation.

BP 80/120 HR ____ Tp 99.2 Rp ____

HT 5' 8" Wt 130 GL ____ Ch ____

Other ______

Diagnosis

Sinus Infection

Actions Needed *(follow-up, referral, prescriptions, tests, etc.)*

	Date Scheduled
1. Perscription for XYZ Antibiotic sent to pharmacy	
2. Follow-up appt in 2 weeks	1/22/XX

Outcome

Treatment started- call if any problems

Web-based Medical Information Resources

Note: You may need to search through some websites to find the specific information you need, but most websites have built-in search capabilities to help you.

Amber Alert GPS System (Individual Locator Device)	www.amberalertgps.com
American Association of Retired Persons (AARP)	www.aarp.com
American Cancer Society	www.cancer.org
American Dental Association	www.ada.org/public
American Diabetes Association	www.diabetes.org
American Foundation for the Blind	www.afb.org
American Heart Association	www.americanheart.org
American Medical Association	www.ama-assn.org
Department of Health and Human Services & Center for Disease Control & Prevention	www.hhs.gov www.cdc.gov
Eldercare Locator	www.eldercare.gov
National Association for the Deaf	www.nad.org
National Hospice & Palliative Care Organization	www.NHPCO.org
National Institutes of Health & National Library of Medicine On-line Service of NIH	www.nih.gov www.nlm.nih.gov www.medlineplus.gov
National Mental Health Information Center	www.mentalhealth.samhsa.gov
National Organization on Disability	www.nod.org
Web MD (General Medical Information)	www.webmd.com

Add your own

Template Pages

Photocopy Masters
Do Not Write on These Copies

Healthcare Concern/Questions/Symptoms

Date ____________

Staple physician's or other healthcare provider's business card or write in contact information here.

Referred by:

____

Include relevant measurements as medical personnel complete your evaluation.

BP ________ HR________ Tp________ Rp________

HT________ Wt________ GL ________ Ch ________

Other ______________________________

Diagnosis

Actions Needed *(follow-up, referral, prescriptions, tests, etc.)*

Date Scheduled

Outcome

Healthcare Concern/Questions/Symptoms Date ____________

Staple physician's or other healthcare provider's business card or write in contact information here.

Referred by:

____

Include relevant measurements as medical personnel complete your evaluation.

BP ________ HR________ Tp________ Rp________

HT________ Wt________ GL ________ Ch ________

Other ______________________________

Diagnosis

Actions Needed *(follow-up, referral, prescriptions, tests, etc.)* Date Scheduled

Outcome

Wallet Card

Instructions: *Photo copy card back to back for 2-sided card*

Complete the wallet card information below and cut out to carry in your wallet for a quick reference. If additional space is needed, make a second card from the template and fold together with the one provided. Review and update information annually or anytime your information changes. Card stock is recommended, but not necessary, for durability.

FRONT

CUT OUT — FOLD HERE — FOLD HERE

MEDICAL INFORMATION

Pharmacy: ____________________

Phone: ____________________

Surgeries: ____________________

____

____

____

Allergies: ____________________

____

____

Eye Glass/Contact Perscription:

____

Blood Type: ____________________

PHYSICIAN INFORMATION

Physician: ____________________

Phone: ____________________

Physician: ____________________

Phone: ____________________

EMERGENCY CONTACT:

Name: ____________________

Address: ____________________

____

____

Phone: ____________________

POCKET REFERENCE

Personal Healthcare Record

Don't Forget

Name ____________________

CONFIDENTIAL

If found, please return to Emergency Contact

Wallet Card
(Note: Photo copy card back to back for 2-sided card.)

BACK

MEDICATIONS	DOSAGE	TIMES/ DAY	DATE STARTED	CONDITION

INSURANCE VERIFICATION FORM

Name of Healthcare Professional ______________________________

Business/Clinic Name ______________________________

Address ______________________________

City/State/Zip ______________________________

Phone ____________________ Email ____________________

The above healthcare professional is responsible for verifying the insurance coverage accepted by his/her office and notifying the patient, in advance of providing services, if the charges will not be covered or are greater than the reasonable and customary charges accepted by the patient's insurance company. The patient will not be held responsible for any charges not communicated prior to services.

____________ ______________________________

Date Signature of Healthcare Professional

SYMPTOM/HEALTHCARE EVENT JOURNAL

(Optional supplement to journal page for detail of major healthcare events or diary of symptoms and responses to treatments.)

Personal Healthcare Record

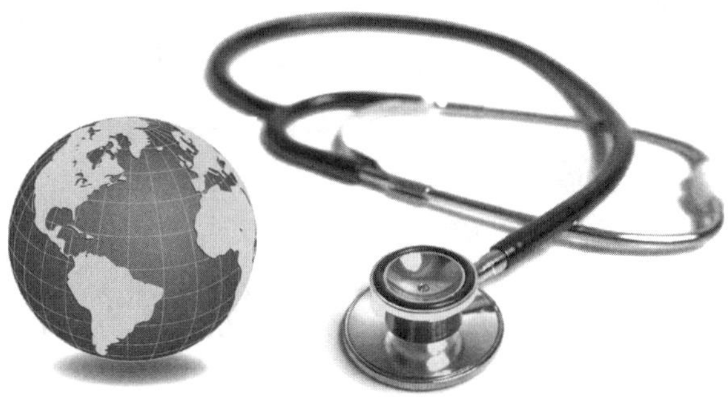

Adult

For ______________________________
Name

From ____________ *to* ____________
Date *Date*

CONFIDENTIAL

Don't Forget

Note: The templates, on the previous page and this page, are to be copied for additional 3 ring view-type notebook inserts, if needed.

Don't Forget

Personal Healthcare Record for: ______________________ *From* ______ *to* ______